PRAISE FOR JASON ANDREWS

"Social anxiety minimal . . . it just evaporated."

—**Jayant G.**, Hong Kong

"Amazing how effective this worked . . . my relationship with my father has healed on a level I consider miraculous. Completely changed."

—**Kyle U.**, New York

"Subject: Promotion & Raise. I got it today! The one I was persuading for!"

—**Rick W.**, Maryland

"I feel really great . . . I really have no desire to check social media."

—**Jaclyn J.**, Kentucky

CHANGE YOUR PAST, CHANGE YOUR LIFE

Author's Note:

I wrote this book not to convey conscious understanding, but to actually change your life experience. This book delivers that change through carefully structured language patterns, in a way similar to what I do for my live clients. In a very real sense, it serves as a kind of "mini session in a book."

Hypnosis works directly with the subconscious mind which, by definition, is outside of conscious awareness. That means that *as you read, the real work is being done "under the hood" at the subconscious level, which you might or might not be able to consciously detect.*

So to get the most out of this book:

1. *Use the 1 to 10 scale I describe in the first chapter if you want to measure your level of change* because that allows conscious tracking without disrupting the subconscious processing

2. *Read this book end to end in one sitting* because it has been designed to work best that way. It should take no more than an hour.

3. *Read this book more than once* because each time you read it, more work will be done at the subconscious level.

CHANGE YOUR PAST, CHANGE YOUR LIFE

Reshape Your Memories, Find Emotional Freedom, and Become Who You're Meant to Be

JASON ANDREWS

This book is for informational purposes only. It is not intended to provide professional advice or to address all circumstances that might arise. Individuals and entities using this document are encouraged to consult their own counsel. The author and publisher specifically disclaim any and all liability arising directly or indirectly from the use of any information contained in this book.

Change Your Past, Change Your Life copyright © 2021 by Jason Andrews

All rights reserved. No part of this book may be used or reproduced in any manner whatsoever without written permission of the publisher, except in the case of brief quotations embodied in critical articles or reviews.

ISBN: 9798745427350 (paperback)

Imprint: Independently published

To P. L. Never underestimate the power of a supportive woman in your life.
To my ancestors. I hope this book makes you proud.
To my descendants. May you use this to be well for seven generations.
To Scott Adams, who in so many ways made books like this possible.

Contents

Chapter 1
Change Your Past, Change Your Life 1
   Why This Works When Standard Therapy So Often Doesn't 4

Chapter 2
How to Alter the Past 7
   Three Steps to Change Your Past and Change Your Life 11
      Step 1 Reshape Memories 11
      Step 2 Experience Emotional Freedom 12
      Step 3 Become Who You're Meant to Be 13

Chapter 3
Case Study: Overcoming Social Anxiety. 17

Chapter 4
Case Study: Releasing Generational Trauma 25

Chapter 5
Case Study: Feeling Safe Again 31

Chapter 6
Changed Past, Changed Life 41

Epilogue 43

Acknowledgments 44

About the Author 45

CHAPTER 1

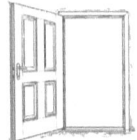

Change Your Past, Change Your Life

Do you ever feel like you are underperforming in some area of your life? Like something is holding you back? What would it be like if you unleashed your real potential? These days there are all kinds of problems that introduce struggle into our lives. Like the epidemic of social anxiety. Everybody who has had parents knows that a lot of internal conflict arises from the process of growing up. And many people have suffered some real trauma. These problems sometimes cause people to feel like things aren't going to get any better. And it's not like you haven't tried to fix things. Very serious people may have told you it's a chemical imbalance, or you were born this way, or suffering is the nature of life, or just go out into nature and exercise more. Some of this advice you took more seriously than others. Maybe you started exercising and ate better, and that helped, but something is still gnawing at you, dragging you down.

And you feel like it shouldn't be.

Well, you're right. It shouldn't be. This book will help you dissolve what drags you down, release what holds you back, and step into the life of effort without struggle.

Specifically, we'll be resolving the past experiences that turn your positive effort into a conflicted struggle.

What do I mean by resolving the past?

This book isn't about changing your past by erasing your memories or inviting you to live a delusion. It's altering the way your problematic memories are encoded in your mind so they don't bother you anymore.

How will you know a memory is resolved? When that memory stops distorting your behavior, your thoughts, and your feelings. So, as you read this book, if certain past situations come to mind that have distorted your own emotions and behavior, that's OK. You may find yourself processing those situations in the same way as my clients in the case studies do. And if *you really do desire to resolve those situations in positive ways*, you might do what my clients do.

As an example, one client of mine had social anxiety stemming from his first day at a new school in junior high. We changed how he experienced and interpreted the event so the pain and confusion went away. He learned what he needed to learn from the situation, and

Chapter 1 - Change Your Past, Change Your Life

that enabled him to move forward in his life with confidence and clarity.

"Social anxiety is minimal. It just sort of . . . evaporated," my client said. He had not talked—really connected—to anyone before because his entire life had been bound up in anxiety. In a few sessions, it was gone. All gone.

How did I know the problem was truly solved? My client then asked me how to talk to people. His social interactions had been so bound up with anxiety that he needed to learn how to talk to other humans. We permanently solved his root problem, and we moved on to the next thing.

Now, many will say that kind of change is impossible or that it takes many months of session work or that invasive pharmaceutical intervention is the only solution. I'm here to tell you that it *is* possible—and quickly. Because when you have the right process or technology, you can make changes that seem like miracles.

So how does it work?

All your memories are encoded in your mind. By adjusting how you store them in your mind—your subconscious mind, specifically—the memories change. Your brain structure changes. Everything downstream is affected. Emotions, behaviors, persistent contexts that inform every thought and decision of life. Your entire life can change.

And that's why conventional therapy so often doesn't work.

Why This Works When Standard Therapy So Often Doesn't

One reason standard therapy fails is that the conscious mind usually doesn't account for the root reason. Your grandmother took your blankie when you were four? A parent said something offhand, not knowing you were in the room? It's hard for most people to accept the irrationality that such a seemingly trivial event can change the course of your whole life. But of course, we know that it can.

Another reason therapy fails is that it's often run by people who are in therapy themselves for unresolved issues. They don't know what a whole, healthy, integrated human looks like, sounds like, feels like. Is it better to learn entrepreneurship from a business school professor or an actual entrepreneur?

Another mistake of standard therapy is that it often aims for the patient to consciously understand the problem. But that doesn't actually solve the problem. In many cases it even makes the problem worse by mentally locking them in to having it for the rest of their life. Have you ever met someone who understands their mental or emotional issue completely . . . but still has the problem? They "buy into" having the problem, and, ridiculous as it sounds, they may even start to defend their problem against attempts to resolve it!

Chapter 1 - Change Your Past, Change Your Life

Crazy, right?

Hypnotists realize that both the root of the problem and the means of its resolution lay in the *subconscious mind.* So that's where we address it. Conscious understanding is optional, and in some cases is actually an impediment.

I'm going to say this again because it's important: *in hypnosis, and in this book, conscious understanding of the process is optional to getting better and to getting good results in your life.* I often ask clients, "Would you rather know what I'm doing, or would you rather get the results you want now, and figure it out later?" The clever ones choose results.

So as the changes happen for you subconsciously - by definition outside of your normal awareness - how can you tell how things have changed? It's important to recognize how much things have changed, so as you read each case study, if your mind can assess how distressful your own situation or event was — say on a scale of 1 to 10 — you can check it again at the end of the book. So that way you can know just how much your life is improving now.

Much has been made recently of cognitive-behavioral therapy, which aims to "re-route" a problematic response into a new behavior without resolving the underlying issue at the subconscious level. Functionality may improve, but the subconscious mind remains dissatisfied with such work because the root cause hasn't been addressed. Many times the mind simply finds a new way to express the issue in an attempt to get you to address the core problem properly.

But as a hypnotist, I work directly with the subconscious mind every day. Our methods resolve the past so it's not a problem anymore, while also changing present behaviors for the better. You need both—past resolution and present change. Only resolving the root cause in the subconscious mind does that completely.

And that's what this book will do for you. We will reshape your memories so they release the negative emotions holding you back, tying you down, and keeping you imprisoned.

You will be free.

And that's when you start to become who you are meant to be.

If this all sounds too good to be true right now, that's OK. I'll ask you again at the end of this book. Until then, let's satisfy your curiosity.

Here's how it all works.

CHAPTER 2

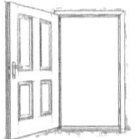

How to Alter the Past

Most people think their memories are real. They think things happened the way they remember them. But did they really? Study after study has shown how unreliable memories can be. For example, DNA evidence has exonerated 375 innocent people in the United States, each of whom served an average of fourteen years in prison based on faulty evidence that often included eyewitnesses who misremembered.[1]

---

1 "Exonerate the Innocent," Innocence Project, accessed April 27, 2021, www.innocenceproject.org/exonerate.

And yet, as every hypnotist knows, the mind often seems to record everything we experience. For example, people hypnotized into a deep trance have been able to recall incredibly specific details about an event accurately—words on a sign in the background or lock combinations and passwords from long ago.

How can both observations be true?

Our minds do seem to archive all raw information deep down. But that's not what we typically access when we remember people, places, things, and events under usual circumstances. What we normally think of as our memories are actually *stored interpretations* of memories. In order to save processing time and brain resources, our minds create and store a summarization of an event for quick retrieval in situations requiring action.

Imagine our caveman ancestors encountering a saber toothed tiger.

"Quick—is that big four-legged orange thing with fangs dangerous or not?" One may have asked himself as a predator approached.

Well, here's a picture of one eating Zog last summer, his brain helpfully supplied.

"OK, thanks, memory. Time to run!"

If our caveman friend had had to recall all the actual details of that earlier situation and reinterpret things anew every time, it might have taken him too long, and he, too, might have met Zog's fate.

Chapter 2 - How to Alter the Past

So our brain is not designed to be accurate as much as it's designed to drive behaviors. In the caveman's case, his brain stored an image that drove the behavior of running away from a predator. Note that his brain didn't provide him with images of saber-toothed tigers grooming each other or lounging playfully because those weren't the images that would have most likely helped keep him alive when he was confronted with one. *One of the mind's key jobs is to protect us, and it's important that it continue to be allowed to happen.*

So our brains evolved to be highly interested in emotional content, particularly anything related to survival and reproduction. And the more emotion embedded in any one memory, the higher the likelihood of deletions, distortions, and generalizations on anything related to that memory. Sometimes those memories get distorted to a degree that they cause real problems, problems you wish could just go away.

When a person gets bogged down with too many memories containing bad feelings, they form a background life context that disempowers them. They may have great difficulty imagining any good things in the future because those bad memories are referenced so often at the subconscious level, resulting in pervasive bad feelings throughout the day.

To change the past is not to rewrite those memories. What we'll be doing is working with traumatic, painful memories—for this sort of memory is always remembered in a distorted fashion, usually in an attempt to prevent the bad thing from ever happening again. To stop reliving the hurts of the past, we'll change how the memory is encoded and, as a result, release the bad feelings embedded in it.

Change enough of those memories, resolve enough of those feelings, and you become a new person. It's as simple as that. And if this seems like a big promise, note that you've actually seen it happen before.

You know how when someone moves to a new city, gets a new job, or lives in a new environment, their life changes? Sometimes their personality does, too. It's because their context changed. The old problems with the old place, job, or home are gone. Their inner world shifts to reflect the new outer world.

We witness a similar phenomenon with people who emigrate from a third-world country or who leave a toxic relationship. They flourish in the new environment primarily because what held them back . . . is gone.

What if you could do this with the context inside your mind? Too many people live in an emotional third world, so to speak, or remain stuck with toxic memories. The big thing in the news these days is a "toxic work environment." Most people's minds are a toxic work environment. Isn't it time to do something about that?

Chapter 2 - How to Alter the Past

THREE STEPS TO CHANGE YOUR PAST AND CHANGE YOUR LIFE

Yes, there are only three. Here's the first one.

STEP 1 RESHAPE MEMORIES

Jonah is twenty-eight years old. He has struggled to connect with people his entire life. No friendship has lasted. He's gone on a few dates. Some were fun. Nothing serious materialized. He tends to be closed off. Because deep down, he suspects no one really likes him.

Jonah came to me when he'd had enough of the loneliness and wanted to do something about it. Through hypnosis, I traced the source of Jonah's issue back to a particular experience he had at the impressionable age of eight. Regardless of the exact age or specific experience, everyone has some event like this, even you. A highly impactful childhood experience.

We revisited the event and had Jonah reexperience those memories armed with the knowledge and understanding of a twenty-eight-year-old adult. His younger self had interpreted what had happened through the limited perspective of a child. That limited interpretation caused Jonah to believe unhelpful things about himself, which continued to affect him long into adulthood.

All we had to do was correct the embedded memory with a proper understanding of that situation. It was as if we "beamed" Jonah's new understanding back to his younger self. In effect, we reshot the scene in his mind.

This change set Jonah free.

A couple of months later, Jonah told me he had started spending more time with some of his coworkers after hours. He was seeing someone now. It was developing into his first serious romantic relationship. He told me that he was still learning how to have friends and how to be a friend because he had never done it before. But he was making progress, and the loneliness was going away.

Through hypnosis, I helped Jonah change his memory, which changed his behavior, which changed his life.

STEP 2 EXPERIENCE EMOTIONAL FREEDOM

Emotional freedom means that the dammed-up emotions within those memories are released and flow away, never to return. Everything downstream from that core event changes. That happened to Jonah. And it can happen to you.

Some hypnosis techniques try to add things to who you are. However, in my experience, you get more from removing what you are not. You are not your fears, injustices, or traumas. You are not your past. The persisting emotions resulting from a painful experience are misleading because the memory was inaccurately encoded to begin with.

Now, when you are reminded of that experience—when you rewatch that movie—it feels entirely different. Because even though you did not literally rewrite the past, you now feel so free that from an emotional perspective . . . you did.

STEP 3 BECOME WHO YOU'RE MEANT TO BE

To become the person you're meant to be, remove everything that is not you. Remove the fears, injustices, traumas, and other distortions, and you begin to feel like yourself again for the first time. You develop an unshakable authenticity, and your choices become more truly your own. Your agency increases. You really do begin to take charge of your own destiny.

You are free. Free to learn. Free to explore. Free to discover the truth for yourself instead of having it filtered through what authority figures have told you. You are improving from "take my word for it" to "let me see for myself."

Take Jonah again. He was told he had social anxiety. He was told he was not neuronormative. He was told that pharmaceutical intervention was likely the only remedy. Otherwise, he would always struggle to make friends, develop lasting relationships, and network for his career.

That made Jonah feel stuck. So he realized he needed to think about himself in terms of what he was doing, which he had the power to change, rather than who he was as a person, which had seemed "baked in" since the day he was born.

Once Jonah got free, his approach to his own experience changed. Instead of relying on old feedback loops—*I'm not normal, so I'm not good with people*—he began to bypass the past and find out for himself what happened when he struck up a friendly conversation. What Jonah discovered was that once that old voice saying that phrase was gone, as if the volume had been turned down to zero, what it had said was actually no longer true. It was only true as long as the voice in Jonah's head was saying it. Saying the phrase had made it true in his experience.

Jonah's reality changed. All the social anxiety he had suffered turned out to be based on a delusion.

When Jonah's memories and accompanying emotions no longer held him back, he was free to start actually experiencing things for himself. So Jonah started at square one, with the basics of talking to other people, like making eye contact and saying hello. And he found that people said hi back. They smiled. Some flirted. At first, Jonah didn't know what to do. But he paid attention to what *he* was doing, and he paid attention to the encouraging responses he got. He used that information to learn how to interact better with people. He had his awkward moments as he made some mistakes, but he learned from them and improved his ability and skill in interacting with others.

"In some ways you're starting from the beginning, but you can test and tweak without the terror," Jonah told

Chapter 2 - How to Alter the Past

me when we caught up a few weeks after our last session. "It's like when you were a kid and learning everything you could and exploring everything you could without any fear. You try something, and if it doesn't work, you get up and try something else. It's amazing to kind of be like a kid again."

Life turned around for Jonah within weeks, not years. And it can for you, too.

Over the next three chapters, we'll cover three life challenges that people commonly ask me for help resolving. We'll run through these three steps to show you how you can free yourself from the past.

CHAPTER 3

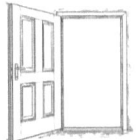

Case Study: Overcoming Social Anxiety

Nigel is from Leeds, England. His father, a biomedical engineer with a background in agriculture, moved the family to Indianapolis, Indiana, for work when Nigel was twelve. Nigel had heard different things about the United States and was both excited and a bit apprehensive to be joining a new school.

"Make a good impression, my boy, so the other children will like you," Nigel's father told him.

Nigel's first day of school was just another day for everyone else. It was the middle of the semester, and

Nigel was the only new kid. That first day, Nigel's English teacher told the class they had a new student and asked him to come up to the front and introduce himself.

"His name is . . . *Nye-gull?*" the teacher sounded out Nigel's name incorrectly as he stood up. The teacher did not have a cosmopolitan background.

Everyone laughed.

Nigel's face flushed.

"How do you do?" he said quietly, in the thickest English accent most of those kids had probably ever heard.

They all laughed again.

"Didn't we beat you in the revolution?" came a voice from the back.

A third laugh followed.

The teacher quieted the class, but it was too late. Nigel had made an impression, but he didn't make a single friend that day.

Fast-forward to when Nigel came to me for help. For close to twenty years, that critical event had fenced in his entire social experience. He was lonely and disconnected. He felt like an outcast with no friends to count on. When we looked into it, I discovered that Nigel had taken his classmates' reaction to mean that he was unwelcome and unlikeable, not just as a new student at a new school but as a person living in the world. Nigel took a sample-size-of-one event in a one-off special circumstance to be true for every social interaction of his going forward.

Middle school and adolescence are challenging times for most people, even under the best of circumstances.

Chapter 3 - Case Study: Overcoming Social Anxiety

Starting at a new school is a stressful experience as well. And Nigel wanted to make his father proud, which added pressure. As we talked further, I realized that Nigel had taken his dad's words and changed them in his mind. What Nigel had heard was, "Make a good impression so the other children will like you," but what he remembered was, "If you don't make a good impression, no one will like you." So I asked him to take that troublesome statement—that problematic belief—and reexamine it with me.

I invited Nigel to notice that the second statement, which he'd kept with him all those years, was not bound by time or circumstance. It was absolute. So to Nigel, it continued to apply—and would do so in perpetuity.

I asked Nigel, "When you think about it now, does that statement have a time component, or does it apply forever?"

Nigel thought about it. He said that although it may have been good general advice, Nigel realized his dad had meant it specifically for his first day of school in America. Then I asked him if there was ever a case when someone didn't make a good first impression, but people eventually liked the person anyway.

Nigel didn't say anything, but I could tell from his facial expression and body language that the belief was beginning to dissolve and that he was seeing some glimpses of what existence could be like without the problem that had dogged him for years.

Then I asked Nigel if he had ever seen *Star Wars*. He hadn't liked episodes seven through nine—they had "rubbed him the wrong way." But he did enjoy the original trilogy and even the prequels.

"When George Lucas made episodes four through six, they didn't have the technology to create the special effects he really wanted. He even created his own company to do the best special effects they could at the time," I said. "But they just didn't have the understanding at the time to do some of the things the way they wanted. However, by the time of the prequels, the people Lucas had hired for episodes four through six had twenty years' more experience and know-how. So after the prequels began production, he had his team go back and reshoot certain scenes with all the understanding and know-how they had gained since then. When George Lucas realized he could reshoot the scenes the way they should have been, he told himself, 'I'm going to *do this now* while I have the opportunity.' And it was a powerful experience for many people to go back and watch the new version of those scenes, which by all accounts turned out better.

"The changes to those scenes also had an interesting downstream effect. Some fan fiction based on some of the old scenes had to be reworked to be consistent with the new timeline. While some things had to be rewritten, the changes opened up a lot of new possibilities for spinoffs, fan fiction, new storylines, and other new content that wouldn't have been possible with the old versions. So there was a bit of disruption, but fairly quickly, the entire baseline world improved."

Chapter 3 - Case Study: Overcoming Social Anxiety

Nigel took a moment to process it all. When he was ready, he said, "You just did something, didn't you? I feel a lot better."

"Yes," I grinned. "I told you about *Star Wars*."

In the days that followed, Nigel told me he had a weird new feeling in social situations. "You know when you need the scissors or something, and you reach into the drawer where you always keep them, but they're not there?"

"Kind of a 'Wait, what?' moment?" I asked.

"Yes, precisely. I feel like that, and, well, I don't quite know what to do."

Nigel had been focusing on his anxiety response in social situations for so long that he had never actually learned how to socialize and to connect with others. We needed to address this.

"So what did you do in your latest social interaction?"

"I watched what others were doing and tried to think of something clever or interesting to say."

"Do people only say clever or interesting things?"

"No, but I want people to think of me as witty."

"Will that make people like you?"

Nigel thought. "No, but it would help," he said.

"Let's start with observing others. Because when you release your need to focus on yourself and start observing others, you begin to notice what they are really saying—both verbally and nonverbally—and that is good information you can use to help you determine what to say and how to say it. Does that make sense?"

"Yes, I believe so. What do I observe?"

"First, notice their body posture and position. Are they slouching? Standing up straight? What are their arms doing? Is their head moving?"

"What does that tell me?"

"Body movements are usually unconscious and are 'tells' for what is going on 'under the hood' in their mind."

"Go on."

"Next, notice their face and facial expressions, particularly those that only last a moment. They give you information as well. And pay particular attention to their tone of voice. Is it loud, soft, strained, relaxed, light, serious? These are all major indicators of what someone is thinking and feeling."

"What about their actual, you know, *words*?" Nigel asked.

"Words don't tell you as much as you might think," I said. "The same words said with a tense body posture and loud tone of voice mean something different than when said with a soft tone and welcoming facial expression. Now, word *choice* does tell you a lot. Did they say, 'I had a hard time with it' or 'I had to fight with it'? That will tell you about their frame of mind and how they view a situation."

"OK, tone of voice, body posture, facial expressions, and word choice. But what do I do with that information? I don't know what those aspects mean when I do notice them."

Chapter 3 - Case Study: Overcoming Social Anxiety

"One thing a lot of good communicators do is they notice one of those aspects of someone's communication and formulate a kind of mini-hypothesis of what it means. Then they think of something that might make sense if that is what it means, and they say or do it. Next, they pay attention to the response they get—tone of voice, body posture, facial expressions, and words—and check if it makes sense according to their understanding of the situation. If it doesn't, they realize they misinterpreted that aspect and generate a new mini-hypothesis to use. If it does, they make note of the new information, and move on to notice a new aspect.

"In this way, over time, you can generate a kind of mental reference library for what aspects mean in different contexts and combinations, to the point where it becomes intuitive to you. Remember when you learned how to ride a bicycle? First, you had to focus on the pedals and the balance and the steering. It was challenging, and you fell down a lot and may have gotten some scrapes and bruises. But did you give up? No, you tried again and again. And eventually you learned the pedaling such that you didn't have to focus much on it—your mind had learned it well enough that it took over the task for you automatically. And then you worked on the balance. And when you got that right, you learned to steer. And from that point forward, the only thing you had to focus on when riding a bicycle was directing it where you wanted to go.

"So now that you understand how that works, you can begin to do that now and from here on out in social situations. And as your skill grows you may eventually find yourself just jumping in on a conversation and enjoying the connection and interaction. As you imagine that now, and look back on today as the start of that process that led you to a skilled and satisfying social life, how does that feel?"

"Bloody fantastic!" Nigel replied in true English fashion.

CHAPTER 4

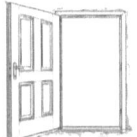

Case Study: Releasing Generational Trauma

Jennifer's parents did the best they could. They strived to treat her and her younger sister fairly. All throughout their childhood, their parents were attentive, compassionate, and understanding. They weren't always perfect, but they tried to make up for when they weren't.

The same year Jennifer graduated high school, the country fell into an economic recession. She had been accepted into her dream university. It wasn't cheap, but she thought she had earned it. But the downturn had hit her family hard, particularly her father, who lost thousands in retirement accounts and had to take a lower-paying job. As a result, the financial support Jennifer had counted on to help pay for college dried up. Her parents explained that their investments had been devastated, and they didn't want to jeopardize their retirement by pulling out any money at the bottom of the market.

"At this point, we can help pay for you to go to a state school, dear, but we just don't have the money right now for a private university," Jennifer's father told her.

Jennifer's grandmother had given her $10,000 toward her education a few years prior. But the market crash had brought that account down to around $6,000. To top it off, the state college's work-study office was overwhelmed with applicants during Jennifer's freshman year, and her parents "made too much money" for her to be included in the program. That meant she needed high-interest student loans and a full-time food service job to get through college.

Three months after Jennifer graduated, her younger sister Ashley started college. By then, much had changed. Markets had roared back and restored millions of people's life savings, including their parents'. Their dad had pivoted back to his lifelong career path and earned a promotion. So when Ashley was accepted into a small, elite private university, her parents were willing and able to pay for it. What's more, that original $10,000 gift from Grandma—which Jennifer had had to use at a lower value of $6,000—was now worth over $16,000 for Ashley. Ashley put that toward a brand-new car and was

Chapter 4 - Case Study: Releasing Generational Trauma

able to chauffeur friends around town on evenings and weekends because she didn't have to get a job.

Jennifer had done very well in school despite the demands on her time and had landed a high-paying job that would enable her to pay off her remaining student loans within five years. Ashley, on the other hand, ended up on academic probation twice.

"She partied too much," Jennifer said during our first session.

At Christmas during Ashley's junior year, the tension boiled over. Jennifer confronted her parents about how she had had to work her way through a state school while her parents paid for Ashley to party her way into trouble at the private university.

Jennifer's mother said, "But look how you turned out. You're doing just great, dear. We're so proud of you."

"No thanks to *you*!" Jennifer snapped.

Her dad stepped in. "You're overreacting. And you owe your mother an apology. You shouldn't complain because we still paid a lot of money to help you through state school. Be happy you got anything because a lot of parents don't pay anything for their kids' school."

"That's complete bullshit!" Jennifer yelled and stomped out of the room.

"Well, it *was* complete bullshit," Jennifer told me years later.

Since college, Jennifer had had some relationships, but her career seemed to always come first. "I don't even really know why," she said. "I'm debt-free and own my own apartment, but the job just doesn't do anything for me anymore. I feel kind of empty."

"And your sister? How is she doing now?" I asked.

"She's a stay-at-home mom with three kids and a rich husband. They met at school."

I could see it in her face. That one hurt.

"What good things are blocked off by that painful event?" I asked her.

I watched Jennifer go inside and discover what was there. "A family of my own," she said quietly.

"It's OK to want that."

I realized that Jennifer had always really wanted a relationship and a family of her own, and that painful experience with her family had kept her from what she had truly wanted all these years. What Jennifer had taken away from that one experience was that she couldn't count on family. So, not surprisingly, her career—and relying on herself emotionally and financially—had always come before even the possibility of having a family of her own. Her desire to have a husband and children didn't go away, but every time she felt that desire, it had been overwhelmed by anger at her parents and resentment of her sister. So Jennifer had buried that desire deep to try to stop the pain.

"How would your life be different without that pain?" I asked.

She started tearing up. "I wouldn't be lonely. I would have someone."

Chapter 4 - Case Study: Releasing Generational Trauma

"What didn't you understand then—at that critical, painful moment—that if you had understood it, things would have turned out better?"

Jennifer thought hard about this.

"Maybe that my parents were embarrassed and ashamed that they weren't able to help me the way they had promised, and they dealt with that the best they could."

"Do you think the way they treated your sister was maybe a way to make up for their inability to provide for you? That perhaps they felt so bad about how little they were able to do for you that they overcompensated with Ashley? Like maybe she was their shot at redemption?"

Jennifer was overcome.

"Now that younger Jennifer's understanding of that situation has changed, how are things different between that event and the present moment? Because they have changed for the better, have they not?"

I let Jennifer sit quietly for a few moments and process the changes. When she was done, I said, "Take a deep breath in . . . and let it all go now." Which she did.

"I feel like I've wasted so much time. I hated my sister for so long for having just been given what I really wanted. But now I realize that everyone did the best that they could with what they had to work with at the time."

"It's OK to change your life now to align with what you truly want," I said. "And you may discover that what truly fulfills you can be different from what you used to think it was or what you were told it should be."

"It's not too late?"

"The best time to plant a tree is thirty years ago," I said. "The second best time is *now*."

CHAPTER 5

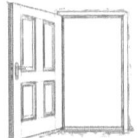

Case Study: Feeling Safe Again

Josef had a fear of wide open spaces. He came to me for help.

"Sometimes I can't even drive by myself on the highways," he said. "It just gets to be too much."

Josef was successful in a number of ways. He had a good job, a house of his own, and healthy relationships with family. But he drank too much, had let himself get out of shape, and had not dated in a long time.

"What am I going to do? I can't drive to pick her up," Josef said. "What woman wants a guy like that? They want someone who is confident. That's not me."

"Yet," I said. "But things can change. How long has this been going on?"

"I've had that sense for about ten years now. It's been depressing to say the least." Josef took a sip from his Starbucks thermos.

"How much coffee do you drink each day?" I asked.

"Two Starbucks ventis," Josef said. "That's the largest size they have."

"That seems like a lot. Are you tired a lot?"

"No. But it keeps the hangovers at bay."

"How much alcohol do you drink?"

"I mean . . . I get drunk like two or three times a week. It's not like I drink every day or anything. I know my limit. I know where you're going with this. I'm not an alcoholic. I quit for a month earlier this year."

"Then why do you drink?" I asked.

Josef thought about this. "Self-medicating, I suppose."

"Are there downsides to it?"

Josef sighed. "Yeah, the hangovers suck. That's what led to the coffee."

I asked a few more questions. I learned that Josef had alternated between depression and anxiety for much of his adult life. He drank to counter the anxiety, which just made the depression worse. Then he overloaded on coffee to jolt himself out of the hangovers and the lethargy. What Josef didn't know was that caffeine drives anxiety.

Like many people, Josef didn't like to be told what to do.

Chapter 5 - Case Study: Feeling Safe Again

"Let me tell you a story," I said. "I was sitting in the waiting room at the chiropractor, and the receptionist was chatting with one of the patients. She had just brought in a drink from the coffee shop next door. The receptionist said, 'Thank you. I love coffee. I drink four cups a day.' 'Four cups a day?' I said. 'If I had that much caffeine, I would either have a heart attack or a panic attack.' Upon hearing this, the receptionist froze and looked off into space. Then quietly to herself, she said, 'I wonder if that has anything to do with it.'"

Josef nodded. I waited for him to say something. He didn't. He nodded some more.

"I didn't bring up the ten dollars a day and the loads of empty calories the coffee was costing her. Caffeine is different from alcohol. Everybody knows the effects alcohol has on you. It's a depressant. Alcohol literally depresses you. You don't like things that depress you, do you? Because feeling depressed sucks, doesn't it?"

Josef looked down and said slowly, "I'd give almost anything to get rid of it."

"What if you could get paid and look better while getting rid of it?"

"What do you mean?" Josef asked.

"How much do you spend on alcohol per week?"

"Two or three six-packs, so I don't know . . . maybe twenty."

"And how much do you spend on coffee every week?"

"Oh, about four bucks each . . . times twice a day, so . . . thirty or forty dollars? Holy shit . . ."

"Let me get this straight," I said. "You spend fifty to sixty dollars every week for the privilege of feeling more anxious and depressed? That's more than two hundred dollars a month. Two thousand four hundred dollars a year to make yourself feel bad."

Josef looked stunned.

"When you think about it like that, it feels like a waste of money, doesn't it? You would get better results by throwing it away because then you wouldn't be adding fuel to the anxiety and depression. You want to get rid of the things that cause anxiety and depression, don't you?"

"Two or three six-packs, so I don't know . . . maybe twenty dollars."

"The first thing you need to do is put that money back in your pocket," I said. "Because you can think of better things to do with twenty-four hundred dollars a year, can't you? I know I can. I now want you to think of three things you can do with that money instead of using it to worsen the anxiety and depression."

Josef thought about it.

"Now imagine a time in the future, facing a situation where, in the past, you would have reached for coffee or alcohol." I paused. "But this time, I want you to watch as future you stops—sees the image of the drink turn black and white—and remembers the things he really wants to spend that money on. Watch as future you pushes the drink away to spend his time on doing something more productive."

I watched as Josef tried this with several different scenarios. "I feel different," he said.

Chapter 5 - Case Study: Feeling Safe Again

"I bet."

In our second session a week later, I asked Josef about his progress. "So how was your week?"

"I still have a six-pack in my fridge, but every time I look at it, I just start thinking about how good it would feel to spend that alcohol money on a trip to the beach . . . the warm, salty air . . . the sound of the waves . . . water as far as I can see . . ."

Josef smiled. I could tell he was at the beach, enjoying himself.

"When I really think about it, the drinking has just lost its luster. It's kind of cold and gray."

"How have you felt this week?" I asked.

"A lot more even. Fewer dark places, more getting out and about."

"And the coffee?"

"Down to one a day."

"It's a process," I said. "How's the anxiety level?"

"Baseline is a bit better. I don't feel as jittery. Sleep is a little better, too. I still can't drive out on the open highway, though—I tried last weekend."

"Let's address that now," I said.

Then I began.

"One of the interesting things about the mind is that, when you consider how well humans learn, we often learn things a bit too well. A certain intense experience can often cause somebody to learn something that is very hard to unlearn later, even though our understanding increases over time.

"So one of the interesting things about my job is that I get to help people change negative things they learned early on that just aren't true. When you go inside and really consider what the source of the issue is—because *your mind does know* what it is—your mind also knows when it started. Your mind knows what happened at that time. So when you go inside and really understand what event it is, now we can begin to make some changes that are going to help you feel better now and in the future.

"Sometimes as you consider an event in the past and what you may have learned from it, you might understand that, at the time, you didn't have the level of understanding that you do now. There's a difference between the way you understand that experience now, and the way you understood that experience back then. If we had understood things perfectly the first time we went through the experience, wouldn't that be great? Well, it's never too late to do that.

"So as you consider that event and what you took away from that event,and how that may have negatively affected you, perhaps you decided that the world was a certain way, or that you had a particular trait or characteristic. Because you didn't have the full understanding back then to know that people change. People learn, people grow, and people change. With the perspective of wisdom that you now have, it's possible to come up with an understanding that would have helped things turn out a lot better, can't you? So you can take a moment to select a particular understanding you lacked then but

Chapter 5 - Case Study: Feeling Safe Again

which would have helped things turn out better back then if you had known it.

"So now that you have that better, fuller understanding, wouldn't it be great if you could go back and tell yourself that fuller understanding, so it was available to you before that event happened? If you do that now you could really change things. Because that understanding would really help you get better takeaways from experience. So as you do that and notice how things change, you might suddenly notice how you feel differently in your body. Things feel different because things have changed, haven't they? Changed for the better. And because this was an event from a long time ago, sometimes other things change—maybe things downstream from that event—and so other things in your past get better, too, because those other things are no longer bound by an incorrect understanding from before. Now they are more open and clear.

"That's a much better perspective. And so as you allow everything downstream to change that needs to change, even all the way to the present moment, you might even look to the future and notice, *wow* . . . even some things in the future may have already changed. Your future may look brighter. You might see more possibilities. You might watch as you see yourself doing things that you always wanted to do but didn't think you could before now. Any voices you may hear are more helpful and supportive. Things *feel better*. Maybe you have new people in your life. Maybe you have better relationships with the people who are already in your life now. Maybe your financial situation has improved. Maybe your health has improved. Whatever it is, as you notice those changes and how good you feel when you see them, you can bring all of those good things back, back into yourself now, and remember how good things are going to be in the future. And when you're ready, you can let me know by nodding your head yes. And you can start that good feeling now."

Josef sat and stared as his mind processed things. I waited.

"Well, it sort of . . . if you . . . I mean, it kind of . . ." Josef grinned. "Yeah."

I smiled, too.

"You may need a good night's sleep for your mind to integrate all these changes fully. Because you have made some good changes, haven't you?"

Josef's grin widened and brightened. "Yeah."

"If you don't want them, we can always change things back."

Josef's face darkened. "No. No way."

"So you want to keep them?"

"Absolutely."

"That's good, because you can certainly do that. In fact, things may even continue to get better."

The next time I heard from Josef, he told me he'd tested driving on the highway with his father beside him. He was able to drive calmly and safely.

"That was a game changer," Josef told me.

That was the change that gave him the confidence to step up and take charge of his life. He had quit drinking altogether and was down to one half-caf coffee a day. He had also dropped fifteen pounds from getting rid of the empty alcohol and coffee drink calories.

"The emotional spikes and crashes are gone," he said. "And that's really kept me on a more even keel. But the real game changer has been the open spaces. I can go anywhere I want now. And there's nothing holding me back."

Josef started driving for a rideshare company on the weekends to practice his social skills and meet new people. One of these customers, a young woman who had just moved to the area, invited Josef to her party. He accepted. As the party wrapped, he invited her out for coffee and a hike. Josef bought them both a decaf and led the way to a nearby park.

They went to a beautiful place that was wide open.

CHAPTER 6

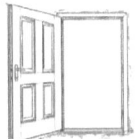

CHANGED PAST, CHANGED LIFE

Most of my hypnosis clients report results like Josef's. They feel free. The chains have been broken. They feel more in control of their lives now. They see opportunities that they hadn't seen before.

Hypnosis works by getting your mind to work with you, not against you. People are often amazed when they realize just how much better their lives can become through a few short conversations with a professional hypnotist.

Jonah, Nigel, Jennifer, and Josef all faced different challenges in their lives. But all their challenges stemmed from emotionally charged events in their past that distorted their feelings and behaviors from that point on. So, using hypnosis, I was able to re-encode those experiences to stop the distortions so they could move forward in their lives with more freedom and choice. We reshape their memories so they experience emotional freedom and become who they are meant to be.

When Josef told his date how he used to be, she asked him, "How did you turn things around?"

"Well, " he began. "There was this book by this guy named Jason Andrews . . ."

Epilogue

As you think back through your experiences reading this book, if you notice that your own past seems to have changed in positive ways, and perhaps you now look towards the future and see a brighter, more open future, with more possibilities and more paths forward, consider sharing this experience in a review. You may also want to revisit that 1 to 10 scale I talked about in the first chapter and notice how much that number has changed now. This book may be a worthwhile read for a friend or family member. And each time you return to the book and read it again, your clarity and understanding will continue to improve, so feel free to do that as well.

I have recorded some hypnosis audio tracks to help others with some specific issues such as relaxation, eating better, and enjoying the experience of exercising. The tracks are available at https://jasonandrews.gumroad.com.

And if you recognize the value in individual sessions, where we can address your specific situation, I made it easy to schedule video time with me from anywhere in the world at http://JasonAndrews.coach/solutions.

Acknowledgments

First off, I would like to thank my editor for helping me make this book a reality; my mentor for helping me resolve my own past and issues; my family for showing me the power of unconditional love and commitment; my clients for being willing to take a chance and reap the great rewards of psychological integration; the great hypnotists, priests, shamans, healers, and others throughout history who have discovered and rediscovered these methods in their own epochs; and the innumerable helpers and effective lieutenants who made things happen for me behind the scenes. And finally, those misguided ones who scrambled my head up so badly in the first place, which forced me to seek out the new methods of restoring wellness that I now bring to others.

About the Author

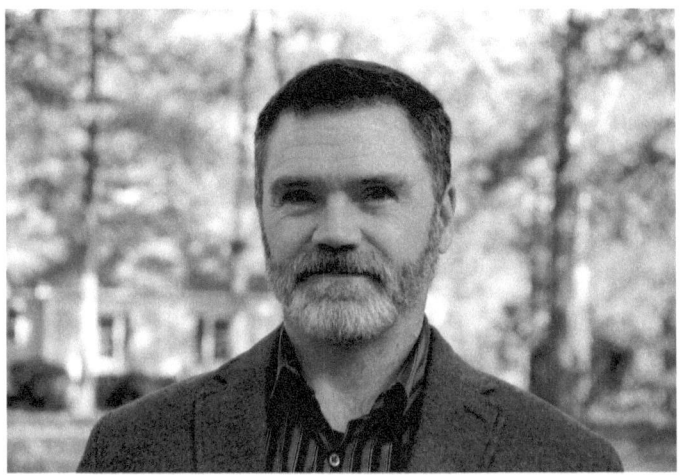

Jason Andrews is a hypnosis-based coach who unlocks potential. Jason is highly praised and often recommended to help clients drop bad habits, be more effective, and find contentment in as little as one session. Learn more about Jason and his work at www.JasonAndrews.coach.

www.ingramcontent.com/pod-product-compliance
Lightning Source LLC
Chambersburg PA
CBHW030511220526
45464CB00006B/2744